# Yoga Beyond the Poses

## *Raja*
# YOGA

*The Ultimate Beginner's Guide
to Discover Patanjali's Yoga Sutras,
Yoga Philosophy, and Meditation!*

*Shreyanada Natha*

*Cover & design*
**Mattias Långström**

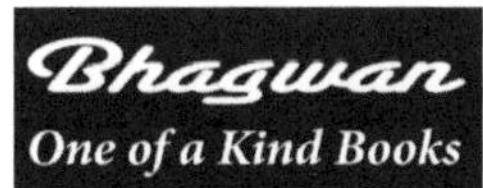

# YOGA BEYOND THE POSES

# Raja YOGA

*The Ultimate Beginner's Guide
to Discover Patanjali's Yoga Sutras,
Yoga Philosophy, and Meditation!*

*Shreyanada Natha*

ISBN 9789198839234

✳ ✳ ✳

# 2 FREE PREMIUM BONUS!

*#1. Download the **AUDIOBOOK** at the back of the book!*

*#2. Download **CHAKRA-INDEX IN COLOR** here!*

*SCAN QR-CODE or go to:*

*https://bit.ly/47wdFVZ*

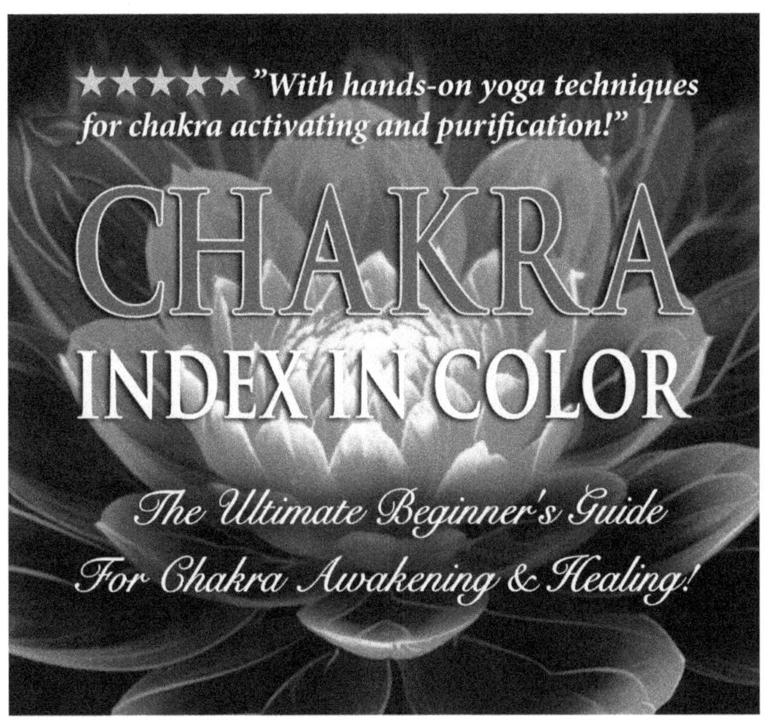

# FREE PREMIUM Audiobook
## Authentic Yoga Nidra Meditation – Mooladhara Chakra Awakening!

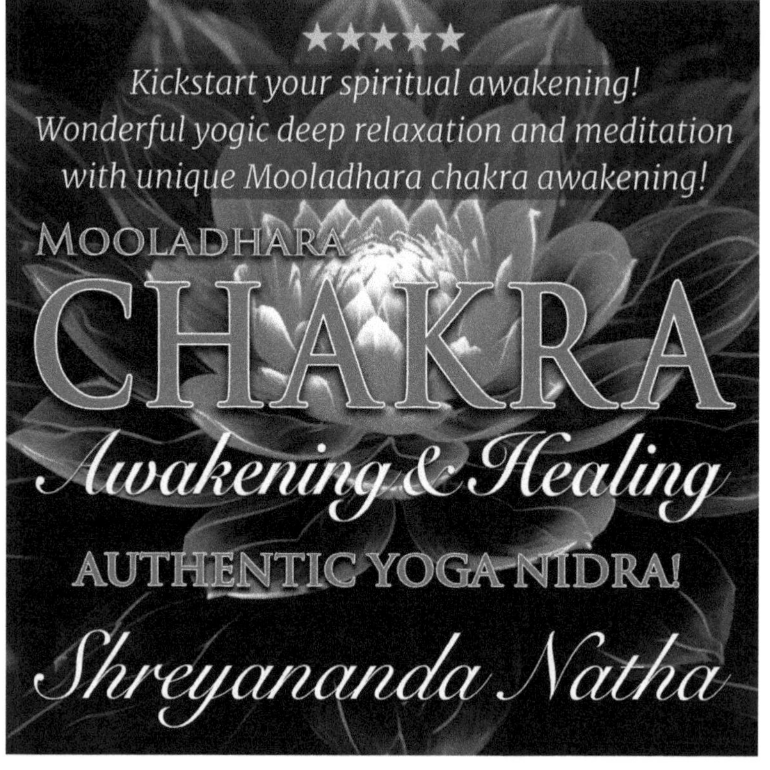


*Download the **AUDIOBOOK** at the back of the book!*

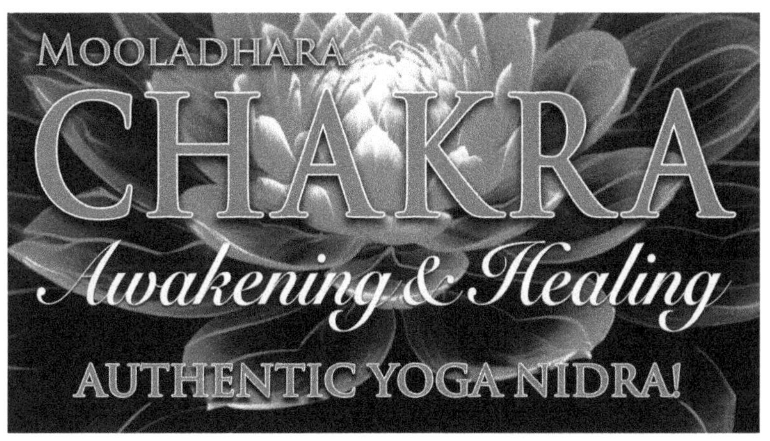


*Kickstart your spiritual awakening! Wonderful yogic deep relaxation and meditation with unique Mooladhara chakra awakening and healing.*

**PRESENTATION**

*Yoga Nidra, or yogic sleep, is a unique meditation process that's powerfully profound and healing for body, mind, and spirit.*

*Practitioners are led into a state of deep relaxation and the experience of our chakra system.*

*Yoga Nidra offers extensive benefits, yet it is one of the most straightforward yoga practices.*

*All you have to do is put on your most comfortable clothes, find a quiet space, lie down on your back, and play the meditation.*

**Yoga Beyond the Poses – Raja Yoga**
**The Ultimate Beginner's Guide to Discover Patanjali's Yoga Sutras, Yoga Philosophy, and Meditation!**
*Including A Premium Audiobook: Yoga Nidra Meditation – Mooladhara Chakra Awakening And Healing!*

*The book describes Raja yoga – yoga as meditation, Patanjali's Yoga Sutras, yoga philosophy, and its origin and mystery from the ground up. It penetrates deeply but remains manageable to read, educational, and comprehensible. A must on the bookshelf for anyone interested in Raja yoga, yoga philosophy, and meditation who quickly wants to know more.*

*The book is part of a series of seven yoga books, Yoga Beyond the Poses: The Ultimate Beginner's Guide to Yoga,  that delve into the seven key areas of yoga.*

**INCLUDING A PREMIUM AUDIOBOOK: AUTHENTIC YOGA NIDRA MEDITATION – MOOLADHARA CHAKRA AWAKENING & HEALING!**
*Kickstart your spiritual awakening! Wonderful yogic deep relaxation and meditation with unique Mooladhara chakra awakening and healing.*

*Yoga Nidra, or yogic sleep, is a unique meditation process that`s powerfully profound and healing for body, mind, and*

*spirit. Practitioners are led into a state of deep relaxation and the experience of our chakra system. Yoga Nidra offers extensive benefits, yet it is one of the most straightforward yoga practices. All you have to do is put on your most comfortable clothes, find a quiet space, lie down on your back, and play the meditation. –*
**Download the audiobook at the back of the book!**

## ABOUT THE BOOK SERIES
**YOGA BEYOND THE POSES:** *The Ultimate Beginner's Guide to Yoga!*

*The book is part of a seven-book yoga series, Yoga Beyond the Poses: The Ultimate Beginner's Guide to Yoga, that delve into yoga's seven most important areas. They are straightforward to read, educational, and fascinating. A must on the bookshelf for anyone interested in yoga who quickly wants to know more.*

## MY NAME AND MY MISSION
*Shreyananda Natha was the name I was given when I was initiated into the Natha Order and received the master mantra – the Shodasi mantra, after studying yoga and tantra for over twelve years, the highest mantra in yoga and tantra. It means "he who knows".*

*After practicing yoga and meditation continuously for over twenty years, having a yoga school for many years, and le-*

*ading studies for yoga teachers, I wanted to get out more wi-
dely with yoga into our whole society, out of the small yoga
room. Spread the knowledge of yoga, our chakra system, and
Kundalini Shakti to anyone who will listen. What needed
to be added were educational fact books on yoga that didn't
just skim the surface or deal with the author's private life. So
it became my Sankalpa, my magical wish, and my mission
to create exciting yoga books that everyone should be able to
read and enjoy. To show how we can apply and use yoga in
different areas of life and achieve success and health. Here
and now.*

*If you like my books, feel free to follow me on my social
media, share and like, tell your friends about the books, and
write an honest review; one or two lines don't matter. All
support is precious.*

*Thanks!*

**THE AUTHOR**

*Shreyananda Natha is the author of popular and best-selling yoga books. He has, among other things, written one of the most comprehensive books about yoga – EVERYTHING ABOUT YOGA and the study book – TEACHING YOGA AND MEDITATION BEYOND THE POSES. He is also a certified yoga and meditation teacher according to the EYTF international guidelines. He has undergone multi-year yoga teacher training under the guidance of Swami Omananda at Satyananda Ashram and holds the highest initiation in the tantric Natha order. He frequently travels to Asia and India to learn and gain knowledge and inspiration. He has immersed himself in tantric rituals and is known for his extensive knowledge of yoga, deep relaxation, and meditation.*

*"There is no authority that can say what yoga is. When you surrender yourself completely and fully and experience yoga without limitations and doubts, the true encounter with yoga occurs when you become one with the true experience within you. Only then will you understand what yoga is – for you. When you are no longer limited by neatness, shyness, and artificial thought patterns that act as a filter between you and the transformation. Yoga is a cultural-historical wealth still passed on from teacher to student and helps man find his way back to his true nature. It opens us up and attracts awareness. It strengthens our self-esteem, and our person's entire spectrum of possibilities suddenly becomes visible.*

*Yoga is not difficult or strange. You don't have to become a vegan, a monk, or be able to stand on your head. You just need to do your yoga regularly; the rest will take care of itself. You can use yoga and meditation to feel better, both physically and mentally, but also to achieve success and develop in all areas of life – here and now."*

*Good luck!*

# NAMASTÉ

*I want to thank the teachers and students I've had over the years who have made my journey with yoga so enjoyable. Thank you for all the inspiration you have given me and for making this book possible. The yoga masters who no longer live among us – live on with each new person who immerses themselves in the yoga tradition.*

*Sri Swami Sivananda, Sri Swami Satyananda, Sri Tirumalai Krishnamacharya, Sri Swami Vishnudevananda, Sri K. Pattabhi Jois, Osho, Swami Nirdosha, Swami Omananda, Swami Janakananda, Ole Schmidt, Turiya, Maryam Abrishami and Sanna Kuittinen.*

*People who all searched for answers to what they sensed through an activated Ajna chakra. In yoga, they have learned the principles behind the universe, the collective consciousness, and the creative force, Kundalini Shakti. The duality behind everything, both what we see and what we don't see. Together, we are helped to pass on the previously secret knowledge about our gunas, nadis, and chakras to all who want to become a Rishi.*

*Aum Shri Durgayai Namaha*

*Shreyananda Natha*

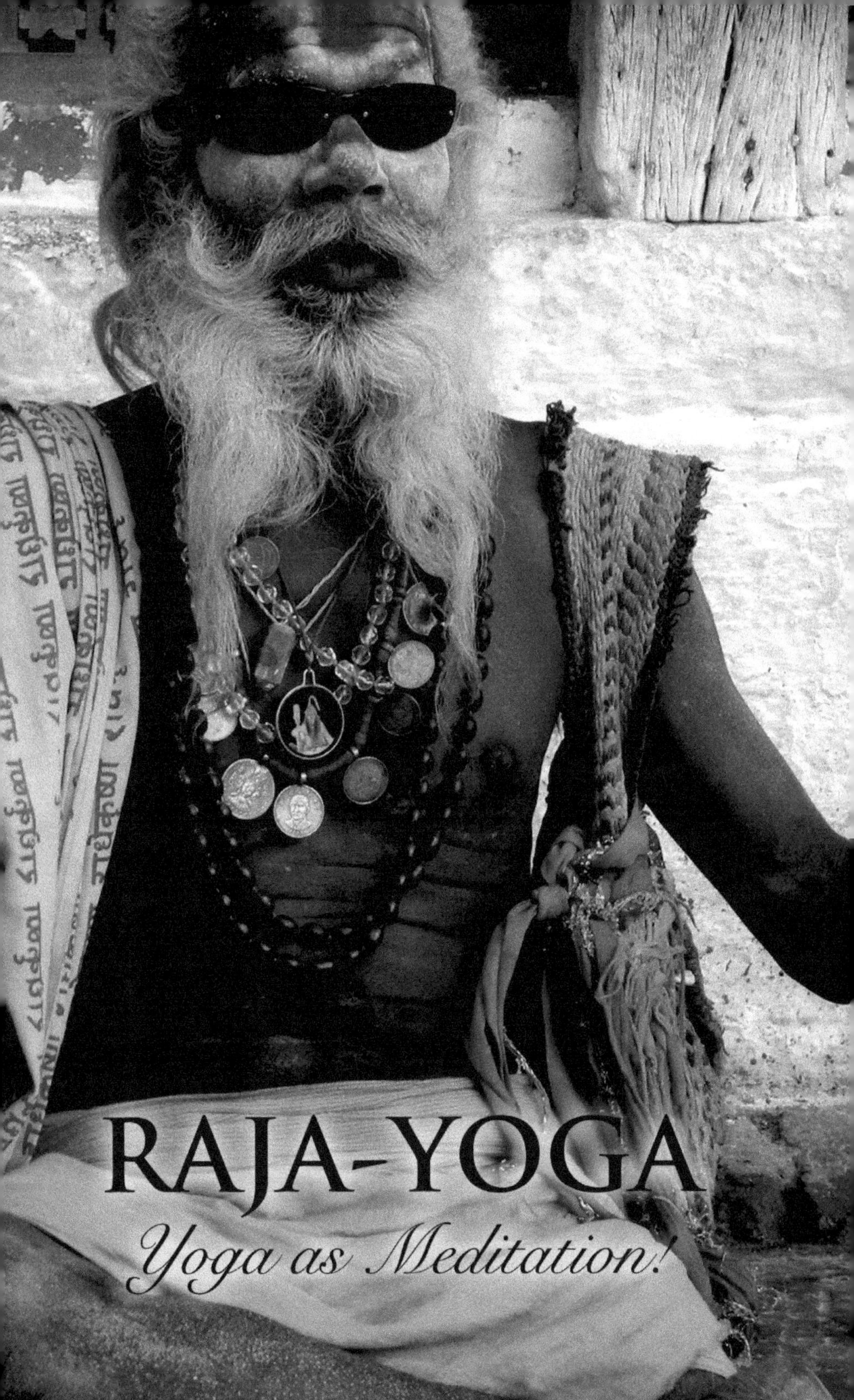

RAJA-YOGA
Yoga as Meditation!

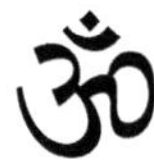

# RAJA YOGA

## SHIVA AND SHAKTI. YOGA PHILOSOPHY'S TWO PRINCIPLES – CONSCIOUSNESS AND ENERGY, MAN, AND WOMAN

## CLASSICAL YOGA & ITS PHILOSOPHY

*In classical yoga and its yoga philosophy, Prakriti (Shakti) is described as cosmic energy. It is the original essence behind everything we can experience, rough and subtle. Prakriti is not in solid form; nothing can be "touched." Prakriti acts as a tool for Purusha (Shiva). Our mind is a result of Prakriti. For consciousness to be able to experience and expand itself, Prakriti is needed. Without Prakriti, consciousness cannot become self-aware.*

*The qualities of Prakriti are what build up our bodies and our world. It carries karma and coexists through which living beings come into existence and shapes our senses.*

*Prakriti consists of three qualities – sattva, rajas, and tamas. These three qualities are a basis for the other elements.*

| **PRAKRITI** | **PURUSHA** |
|---|---|
| *All experiences.* | *The experience.* |

*Manifested.*

*Unmanifest.*

*Background to everything.*

*Eternal subject.*

*Materially and mentally.*

*Infinite amount.*

## THREE PRINCIPLES BUILD A COSMOS

*Thus, our world is built from these three principles – in varying combinations, rajas, tamas, and sattva. The interactions between these gunas govern the cosmos, society, and every human being.*

*Two primary "laws" describe the interaction between these three works. The first is the "law of alternation," meaning they are in constant motion and collaborate. In sattva, rajas and tamas also exist. In rajas, tamas and sattva live and in tamas, rajas and sattva live. They work together all the time.*

*The second is the "law of continuity." By this, it means that when a guna has become dominant, it tends to be so for some time.*

*In yoga, a sattvic state is seen as something of a higher quality, which causes us to develop spiritually. Yoga practice consists of two steps. To create a sattvic condition and then go beyond this condition. This means that we should first purify the body and mind and then go beyond the body and mind and experience our true nature beyond all manifestation. There is also a hidden, mysterious knowledge tradition about activating our chakra system that we will go through later. The fundamental pre-condition for the chakra system to be activated is that the sushumna is open, and that is only when you are in a sattvic state. In scientific terms, these three gunas are described as:*

**SATTVA**
*Pure vibration/balance.*

**RAJAS**
*Movement.*

**TAMAS**
*Inertia / slow / immobility.*

*One talks about three human characters. The guna that dominates us determines what character we have. You should know the different personality traits and adapt the yoga practice accordingly.*

*If you are tamasic or slow, it is good with a dynamic form of yoga where you get the activity going in the body and, in this way, can create balance. Hatha yoga or physical work suits tamasic people.*

*If you are rajasic or mobile, you often need help with concentrating. Here, it is essential to have a lot of relaxation but to relax and release tension, a dynamic form of yoga is also required. You exhaust your body and mind to be able to relax more easily. Hatha yoga, Bhakti yoga (e.g., kirtan), Japa yoga, and Karma yoga suit rajasic people.*

*If you are sattvic or balanced, it is easy to focus and concentrate and well suited to Satsang and studies. But even if you are sattvic, you must work with the body. It's to create balance in the already balanced thought activity.*

*A rule to follow is that inertia is balanced with movement, and movement is balanced with even more movement. We always start with the outer, the surface, our body, and go inward, deeper, balancing and activating. We always start with the movement. Always.*

## ISHVARA

*Yoga is a practical method based on the Samkhya philosophy, but unlike Samkhya, yoga's view of creation is theistic.*

*In classical yoga, the God or creator is called Ishvara in Sanskrit. Ishvara is said to be the force that creates, maintains, and destroys the world through the three forms: Brahma, Vishnu, and Shiva, as well as their female counterparts Saraswati, Lakshmi, and Kali.*

*Although Ishvara is very similar to our Western God, they differ in that Ishvara works through different gods and goddesses; it has different shapes and manifestations. Ishavara can also be worshiped in a female form and is then called Ishvari. It's common in many yoga traditions, especially those of tantric origin. Ishvari is then equated with Shakti.*

*Ishvara is not described separately in Samkhya, but in many yoga traditions, Ishvara is described as Purusha (Shiva in tantrism).*

## DARSHANS

*Vedas are writings composed of rishis (sight/medium) and yogis about 5000 years ago (they can also be much older). These describe the wisdom behind the cosmic mind, which is said to be the origin of the universe and creation. From the beginning, these writings have been passed on orally and then written down. Yoga has its roots in Vedic teachings. Rishis gave Vedic knowledge a practical form, yoga.*

*From the Vedas, six philosophical paths/views were developed, shad darshans, which means "six ways of seeing" or "six ways of insight." Ass described by Patanjali in the Yoga Sutras, classical yoga is one of these.*

*Hiranyagarbha, the sun god, and the cosmic creator, is traditionally said to be the creator of the yoga system.*

*The six Vedic / spiritual paths:*

*1. Nyaya – logical doctrine – Gautama.*
*2. Vaisheshika – atomic doctrine – Kannada.*
*3. Samkhya – the doctrine of the cosmic principle – Kapila.*
*4. Yoga – the doctrine of yoga – Hiranyagarbha.*
*5. Purva Mimamsa / vedanta – ritual doctrine – Jasmine.*
*6. Yttara Mimamsa / Vedanta – theological doctrine – Bada-rayana.*

*Nayaya and Vaisheshka's teachings are based on logical philosophy. These can be compared to Plato's philosophy as we know it in the West.*

*Samkhya is the philosophy behind yoga and Ayurveda. It is based on a scientific approach that explores our inner and outer reality. Samkhya describes tattwas / cosmic principles that one tries to gain insight into and experience with the help of various yogic exercises. Samkhya describes the knowledge behind the different elements, and yoga is a technique that should purify and balance the corresponding components in ourselves.*

*Purva Mimamsa refers to Karma yoga, which acts as a channel for the creative energy of the universe. You work and contribute with selfless services/work to people and society. It is also part of focusing on a prayer or a mantra during the work. It cleanses both the mind and the body and is a good preparation for meditation.*

*Uttara Mimamsa is the system where you go in-depth for the Vedic texts. One discusses God, the soul, the absolute, and their interaction.*

## AUM

*A common symbol in yoga is Om. The emblem is made up of three syllables that together form a whole. Sanskrit's vowel "o" consists of "a + u." So, Om can also be spelled as Aum. It represents the trinity of our existence.*

*The symbol A-u-m consists of three "curves," a semicircle and a point. The most significant "curve" at the bottom refers to our waking state when our consciousness is turned outwards and when we take in the environment with the help of our sense organs. It's called jagarat. It is symbolized by the most significant "curve" because it is our most common state. Beta waves dominate in this state – we are aware.*

*The second largest curve at the top of the symbol refers to deep sleep and our unconscious state. We neither dream nor feel desire. This condition is called sushputi. Delta waves dominate in this state – we are unconscious.*

*The slightest curve between these two refers to our dream sta-*

*te, swapana. Here, the consciousness is turned inwards; you experience the world with closed eyes. Theta waves dominate in this state—the experience of the subconscious.*

*The point in the symbol refers to our fourth state of consciousness which in Sanskrit is called turiya. Here, we look neither outwards nor inwards but are in pure being. That is the unmanifest state of Purusha. Alpha waves dominate in this state – we are superconscious.*

*The semicircle refers to the Maya, which separates the point turiya from the "three curves." Maya symbolizes what hinders our ability to experience our true nature. That the semicircle is just half tells us that Maya cannot change the experience that exists within us, the stillness/being/bliss. Maya can only decide what is manifested.*

*Aum thus symbolizes the manifested and the unmanifested. What we can see and cannot see represents the trinity of our existence. The sound and vibrations that occur when we sound Om / Aum affect our whole being on all these levels and are a powerful mantra. It permeates our entire interior and makes us vibrate in step with the universe. Aum – the sound/vibration of the cosmos and creation.*

**VIVEKA**
*Patanjali (the author of the Yoga Sutras) describes Viveka,*

*i.e., discernment. The purpose of eight-step yoga (classical yoga) is precisely to develop Viveka within us, i.e., awareness, which is a prerequisite for understanding the goal of yoga.*

*It requires a sharp ability to pay attention and distinguish the experiencer from the experience, see what our true identity is and what is perishable. We also need intense attention to know the reason for our ignorance of this – i.e., to miss what is changeable for immutable, to forget what is destructive for improvement, to ignore desires for need, to identify with the ego instead of the true self.*

## VAIRAGYA

*When we developed Viveka, a change took place in us. We begin to let go of our desires. It is called Vairagya. We no longer cling to what will disappear anyway. When we understand the principle of transience, we can take a more understanding approach to life's worries and troubles. If you read about the yoga philosophy, you know that Buddha was enlightened in India at about the same time as Patanjali, where he took his inspiration for the eightfold path. People often talk about Buddhism as a cousin of the yoga philosophy. Many of the ideas are similar.*

## RAGA

*Everything we experience and "take in" from our surroundings happens with our senses. Through our eyes (sight), ears (hearing), nose (scent), tongue (taste), body/skin (feeling), and mind (thoughts, feelings, images). They can then be divided into comfortable, uncomfortable, and neutral experiences. Most often, we want to re-experience the comfortable experiences and provide enjoyment. We want to recreate these experiences time and time again. It is called raga.*

*Events that we experience as painful and unpleasant, we want to avoid. Most of the time, we try to find what gives us pleasure and avoid what is painful. It creates dissatisfaction and a divided mind. We need more than what is. We do not accept life for what it is.*

## DRASHTA BHAVA

*In yoga, we create a third approach called drashta bhava. It can be translated as "witness attitude." Here, we have a neutral and relaxed attitude to our negative and positive thoughts. This approach, with Viveka, leads to liberation, the ultimate purpose of yoga. To be free from desire, not to be controlled by ideas and feelings. To be happy with what is – whatever it looks like right now. To accept what we cannot change.*

## CURRENT CLASSICAL YOGA:

## SATYANANDA YOGA

*Today, classical yoga is taught through, among other things,*

*Satyananda yoga. It is a system developed by Swami Saty-ananda Saraswati. They use ancient and traditional tech-niques: Asanas to balance body and mind, pranayamas to work with the energy body, and meditation to calm and focus the mind. Tradition teaches the general yogic lifestyle to the "ordinary modern man" and the more devoted prac-titioner. Everyone can take part in yoga. Jnana, Bhakti, and Karma yoga, among others, are also part of the Satyanada system.*

*In Satyananda yoga, one considers the whole being of man, not just the body. You want to give the individual an oppor-tunity to discover and develop all aspects of one's personality with the help of yoga. It is believed that change happens with regular practice, under entire presence and awareness, not by pushing the body or mind beyond its means.*

## SRI SWAMI SIVANANDA SARASWATI

*Swami Satyananda's guru and perhaps India's most famous yoga personality – Sri Swami Sivananda Saraswati, was born in Pattamadai in 1887. Sivananda worked as a doctor before quitting to find his guru in the Himalayas. He settled in Rishikesh, where he was initiated into dashnami sannyasa by his guru Swami Vishwananda Saraswati in 1924. Over the years, he and his disciples wrote hundreds of books and articles on yoga and spirituality to spread the knowledge to the general public. Sri Swami Sivananda wanted to give the needy the knowledge that could help them, whether it was about improving physical health, creating peace of mind, or developing spiritually. It still characterizes Satyananda yoga today.*

## SWAMI SATYANANDA SARASWATI

*Swami Satyananda Saraswati was born in Almora in 1923. At nineteen, he met Sukhman Giri, from Juna-Akhara, a Tantric yogini from Nepal. From her, he learned, among other things, the Tantric nyasa techniques, which he developed further with Swami Sivananda. Nyasa is a technique for raising awareness by placing different energies in the body parts. From there, he created the world-famous deep relaxation yoga nidra. In 1943, he met his guru, Swami Sivananda, and was initiated into dashnami sannyasa in 1947. After serving his guru's mission for twelve years, Satyanada began his journey through India as an ascetic to discover the needs of society. In 1956, Swami Satyananda founded the International Yoga Fellowship and, in 1963, the Bihar School Of Yoga, hoping to spread ancient yogic knowledge to all corners of the world. For twenty years, Swami Satyananda traveled worldwide, spreading the wisdom of yoga. He and his disciples also authored over eighty yoga, Tantra, and spirituality books. In 1984 he founded the" Yoga Research Foundation" and "Sivananda Math" to help disadvantaged people.*

## YOGA FORMS

*In Satyananda yoga, the following forms of yoga are applied:*

## JNANA YOGA

*The path of spiritual insight is where one, through intellectual and theoretical knowledge, studies life and tries to distinguish the truth from the perishable. This path is suitable for theoretically inclined people.*

## BHAKTI YOGA

*The path of devotion and love consists of song, dance, or meditation on an image of a guru or the divine. The practicer strives to create a personal relationship with the sacred and merge with it.*

## KARMA YOGA

*Selfless service is where you help others and society without taking advantage of it or shining in the glory.*

## HATHA YOGA

*Here, you want to balance and strengthen the physical and mental body as a preparation for the more advanced exercises in Kundalini yoga. Asanas, pranayamas, bandhas and shatkarmas are used.*

## RAJA YOGA – CLASSIC YOGA

*The path of meditation. It refers to the system described in Patanjali's Yoga Sutras.*

## KRIYA YOGA

*Satyananda taught Kriya yoga based on the secret exercises of yoga and tantra shastras. Kriya means "activity" or "movement" and refers to the natural movement of consciousness. Kriya yoga does not stop the movements of the mind but instead creates an action in the mind that leads to a conscious increase and awakening. There are seventy kriyas, of which twenty are best known and used.*

## THE TRADITIONS

*In addition to the yogic tradition, Satyananda yoga also includes the Tantric and Vedic traditions.*

*Tantra refers to practical exercises that expand the human consciousness and the awakening of Kundalini Shakti. The principle behind the tantric system is that one uses the material world and its experiences to become enlightened.*

*Tantra is often described as a sexual tradition where you want to enhance the sexual experience. Originally, Tantra was intended to awaken Kundalini Shakti, a dormant potential force in man.*

*There are many tantric paths, and the common denominator of these paths is the use of mantras, yantras (concentration symbols used to liberate consciousness), chakras, mandalas (discovering macrocosm in microcosm), tapasya (self-purifi-*

*cation), Raja yoga, pranayama, shaktipat (power transmission) and Tantric initiations to reach awakening.*

*Tantrism advocates a life in which the qualities of the intellect and the heart are exploited. To discern and focus with the help of the mind and to see and experience with the spirit the unseen, the cosmic consciousness beyond the material.*

*The Vedic tradition is one of the oldest preserved spiritual traditions in existence. It advocates the divine as the ultimate truth and life accordingly in the material world.*

*Central to Vedic doctrine is that God is constantly present, omniscient, and omnipotent, while the individual is only an actor. To experience the reality that is Satyam (truth), Shivam (favorable), and Sundaram (beautiful), the individual should live a life where one strives to harmonize thoughts, behavior, and actions: a meditative contemplation, belief in God and oneself. Living in harmony with, and being grateful for, the environment and nature and experiencing unity are the foundations of the Vedic tradition.*

*All the Vedic and Tantric traditions are held together by yoga. Yoga is the practical principle of the spiritual paths that lead to increased awareness and self-insight.*

## RAJA YOGA – THE ROYAL PATH

*Patanjali never gave his system any specific title. He called it yoga. In time, however, his method became known as Patanjali's and classical yoga. Patanjali's yoga is one of the different forms of Raja yoga (Raja means royal):*

*Kundalini yoga (also called Laya yoga).*
*Kriya yoga.*
*Yoga mantra.*
*Dhyana yoga.*
*Patanjali yoga.*

*Raja yoga is the doctrine of the mind. You explore your inner world to exploit your strength and knowledge here. Raja yoga teaches different methods to create a focused mind. It is based on mental discipline.*

*Patanjali defined his method as "elimination of mental fluctuations" – Yoga chitta vritti nirodha. Usually translated to – when the mind is still, yoga occurs. The mind can be described as the visible part of the pure consciousness and divided into the conscious, the subconscious, and the unconscious. Patanjali's definition means yoga is the control of the pattern of consciousness.*

## VIYOGA

*Who is experiencing this?*

*Most people know that yoga means union, but in the Yoga Sutras, Patanjali describes yoga as a separation process. It can be explained by the Samkhya philosophy, which is the foundation of the Yoga Sutras.*

*Samkhya divides existence and individuality into two aspects we have touched on – Purusha and Prakriti. The existence and the individual are created when these two merge. Purusha refers to the one who sees / experiences drashta. Prakriti refers to the seen, drishya.*

*Practicing yoga and its process leads to yoga, a separation between the one who experiences and the seen. It leads to yoga, the association that is the very development of yoga, the culmination. At first, Purusha and Prakriti must be separated from each other, and then it is understood that these are the same.*

*It can also be described that the pure consciousness (Purusha) is broken down by incorrect identification with mind and body (Prakriti). The purpose of yoga is to release pure consciousness from the mind and body.*

*The experience of the difference and separation between Purusha and Prakriti leads to the realization that everything is the same.*

"A METHOD BY WHICH CONSCIOUSNESS IS DISCONNECTED FROM ENTANGLEMENT WITH MIND AND THE MANIFESTED WORLD. YOGA (UNION) IS THE RESULT OF"

**EIGHT STEPS / ASHTANGA**

*Patanjali describes a series of techniques that have a slow and harmonizing effect on our minds and perceptions. The most crucial thing in Patanjali's system is described in the eight steps. The first five steps are preparatory to the other three steps and belong to bhairanga / outer yoga. Ashtanga means eight different steps and should not be confused in this context with the modern Ashtanga yoga developed by yoga master Shri K. Pattabhi Jois.*

*You must not see the first five steps as a staircase; you can also see it as a wheel where you influence others by working with one step.*

*1. Yama – is about moral discipline in social life.*

*2. Niyama – is about restraint on a personal level.*

*3. Asana – sitting position/body position. It refers to the correct meditation position/lotus position so that you can remain immobile during the meditation and are not distracted by the physical body.*

*4. Pranayama – respiratory regulation / control of prana / kumbhaka. By controlling breathing, you can control the life force/prana in the body and calm the mind.*

*5. Pratyahara – removal of sensory impressions. By blocking sensory impressions, one is not distracted by the external environment.*

*The last three steps belong to antharanga / inner yoga. One must have absorbed the first five preparatory steps to develop in-depth and succeed with these steps. The steps before pratyahara gradually dissolve external obstacles in life, while the exercises after eliminating thoughts and inner images so that the mind is still. Ida (our inner world) becomes balanced with pingala (our outer world) so that the sushumna (our supersensible world) begins to exist during samadhi.*

*6. Dharana – concentration. Focus on a meditation object.*

*7. Dhyana – meditation. After a more extended concentration, you naturally sink into meditation. Here, one is fulfilled by the meditation object.*

*8. Samadhi – liberation/ecstasy / superconscious. Meditation eventually leads to samadhi. Here, the movements of the mind have stopped, and you become one with the meditation object and experience powerful ecstasy/joy. There are twelve stages of samadhi; the last stage leads to the liberation of the cycle of rebirth.*

*The eight steps gradually balance our five koshas (shells):*

*Annamaya, pranamaya, manomaya, vijnamaya and anandamaya. The boundary between the shells is loosened from the coarsest – the body, annamaya kosha, to the most subtle, our innermost interior – anandamaya kosha.*

## YAMA

*Satya – truth, to be true to oneself and others.*
*Ahimsa – do not be involved in the killing.*
*Asteya – do not steal, do not take more than you need, and share.*
*Aparighara – not to be greedy, to live materially.*
*Brahmacharya – chastity. To live ascetically, not indulge in pleasures as they are considered to distract one from reaching the goal of yoga.*

## NIYAMA

*Saucha – purity of speech and action, sensory impressions (media, television, radio), food, hygiene.*
*Santosha – contentment, to be happy with what you have. If we focus on what we do not have, we create even more emptiness within ourselves. If we focus on shortages, we get even more shortages (the law of attraction).*
*Tapas – self-discipline, hardening of the inner fire.*
*Swadhyaya – studies.*
*Ishwara pranidhara means to surrender one's will to the higher will.*

*Yamas thus create a balance in our interaction with the outside world, and niyamas harmonize our inner feelings. These rules are designed to balance our external actions with our internal settings. The mind affects our external actions at the same time as our external actions affect the mind. If our actions are not good, the mind will also be negatively affected, which creates a vicious circle as a distracted mind creates less good actions. Yamas and niyamas are designed to break the vicious circle. It can be challenging to follow these rules, but even a small change does a lot to balance the mind.*

"I'M WAITING TO LEAVE THIS BODY, BUT I'M
NOT GOING TO LEAVE IT UNTIL I GET MY
RETURN TICKET. I DO NOT WANT EMANCIPA-
TION, MOKSHA, OR ANY PERSONAL SATISFAC-
TION THAT COMES WITH SPIRITUAL ENLIGH-
TENMENT. MY AIM AND ASPIRATION IN THIS
AND ALL FUTURE LIVES IS TO HELP OTHERS.
TO WIPE THE TEARS OF SUFFERING AND PAIN
FROM THE EYES OF EVERY PERSON SEEKING
SOLACE, PEACE, PLENTY, AND PROSPERITY.
THAT IS THE ONLY PURPOSE OF MY LIFE."

(SWAMI SATYANANDA SARASWATI)

# PATANJALIS YOGA SUTRAS

*Patanjali's work consists of one hundred and ninety-six sutras. The word sutra itself is often incorrectly translated as verse. The actual translation is "to thread in a row," which also describes how the sutras are linked to each other and carry an underlying continuity. The work is considered the most accurate and scientific yogic text ever written.*

*Who Patanjali was and when he lived is still being determined. It has also yet to be possible to decide when his work was written and whether he was a man or a woman. There is still some evidence that he must have lived about 300-400 years BC.*

*Patanjali gives us a range of techniques that gradually balance and harmonize our minds. The unique thing is that Patanjali does not describe a single yoga position as we are usually used to. Here, instead, the focus is on yoga from a moral perspective. When Patanjali talked about asana, he referred to a steady and comfortable position to sit and meditate in.*

*Many great masters and yogis have translated and interpreted Patanjali's work.*

*The following sutras are some of the most important to know:*


**3:2**
*Cause of suffering.*
**Avidyāsmitārāgadveṣābhiniveśāh kleśāh**
*Avidy: erroneous knowledge, asmit: I-experience, raga: liking, dves: reluctance, abhiniveh: fear of death, klesah: suffering.*


*Klesha is the suffering that is present in everyone. According to Patanjali, the basis of all suffering is incorrect identification with the experience. Everyone carries a subconscious suffering, but we are seldom aware of it in our daily lives; all the musts and chores block the experience of it.*


*We rarely become aware of our fear of dying, even if it is in our subconscious. The fear of dying is the basis of our most incredible suffering. Kleshas is like a chain of misfortune that begins with our ignorance of our true nature based on our ego. We try to find pleasure and avoid suffering, creating fear and tension. The solution to being free from suffering is meditation.*

**4:2**

*The root cause.*

**Avidyākṣetramuttareṣām prasuptatanuvichchhin-
nodārāṇām**

*Avidya: incorrect knowledge, ksetram: area, uttaresam: of
the following, prasupta: dormant, tanu: weak, vichchhinna:
alternating, udaranam: fully active.*

*Avidya is the field of dormant, weak, alternating, and fully
active states of kleshas.*

*Avidya is the basis of the other four kleshas: asmita, raga,
dweshta, and abhinivesha. These are either dormant, weak,
alternating, or fully active. When we learn to deal with
avidya, we can also learn to deal with the other four kleshas
more easily. Avidya is about the ignorance of our true nature. We must learn to control the kleshas to return to our true
nature.*

5:2

*Incorrect knowledge.*

**Anityāśuchiduhkhānātmasu nityaśuchisukhātmakhyāti-
ravidyā**

*Anitya: not eternal, asuchi: unclean, duhkha: pain, natma-
su: not atman, nitya: eternal, suchi: pure, sukha: goodness,
atma: self, khyati: knowledge, avidya: erroneous knowledge.*

*Avidya means that one confuses the eternal, impure, and evil
with the infinite, pure, good, and atman.*

*Avidaya is about ignorance of our true nature and identifica-
tion with the body. We are free from Avidaya by developing
our discernment, viveka. Through viveka, we can distinguish
between our body and atman, our inner true self.*

*Avidaya is also called Maya. In a cosmic context, it is called
maya, and on an individual level, it is called avidaya.*

**6:2**

*Separation, I, ego.*

**Dṛgdarśanaśaktyorekātmatevāsmitā**

*Drg: Purusha, the power of consciousness, darsana: the seen, saktyoh: of the two forces, ekatmate: identity, eva: like that, dodge: I-feeling.*

*Asmita can be described as an identification of Purusha as a Buddhi.*

*Asmita means that our inner consciousness, our true self, is mixed with our existence, body, actions, and mind. When our true self is expressed through the body, actions, and mind, it is called asmita. Purusha is identified by its means of expression/instrument. It can be expressed in different ways, as identification with the body or in a more intellectually developed person as identification with the more developed sensory functions. Our ability to see, think, and hear comes from Purusha, expressed through our senses. When we mix these, it is called Asmita.*

*Shakti, the power of Purusha, lies behind the ability to think, see, etc., mixed with the actual means/instruments with which these are expressed. By meditating, we can realize that Purusha is not a part of the body or the intellect (Buddhi). We come across Asmita.*

**7:2**

*Attraction, I want.*

**Sukhānuśayå rāgah**

*Sukha: satisfaction, anusayl: accompanying, ragah: pleasure, liking.*

*Raga is the pleasure created by satisfaction.*

*Raga is about the mind constantly wanting to recreate a previous experience of pleasure.*

**8:2**

*Repulsion, I do not want.*

**Duhkahānuśayå dveṣah**

*Duhka: pain, anusayl: accompanying, dvesah: reluctance.*

*Dwesha is our reluctance to experience pain.*

*Dwesha is the opposite of raga. You want to avoid what creates discomfort. Raga and dwesha keep us in the lower stages of consciousness. As long as raga and dwesha rule over us, we do not develop spiritually.*

*To like something also means you do not want the opposite of what you like. So raga and dwesha are not opposites but two sides of the mind. Dwesha is what affects us most negatively because it is based on a lot of hatred. The elimination of dweshta allows for more profound meditation and the natural elimination of raga.*

**9:2**

*Fear of dying.*

**Svarasavāhī viduṣo ́pi tathārūdho ́bhiniveśah**

*Svarasavahi: persistence of self, vidusah: of the learned, api: also, tatha: like it, rudhah: dominant, abhinivesah: fear of death.*

*Abnivecha is the hope of being able to live and be maintained by one's power, even among scholars.*

*It is the most dominant klesha. All individuals experience fear of dying. It is an innate, inherent force that exists naturally in us, a self-preservation drive. As children, we do not share this the same way, but the older we get, the more aware we become of it.*

*In those who have developed viveka, abhinivecha is almost eliminated. Still, in most people, it can be seen in its most active form, which can also lead to fear and panic in, for example, a severe illness. In ancient Indian texts, one can read about the cause of abhnivecha, which is identifying with the body.*

**11:2**

*Meditation – the solution to the elimination of kleshas.*

**Dhyānaheyāstadvṛttayaḥ**

*Dhyana: meditation, heyah: reduces, tadvrttayah: modification, change.*

*The modification of the kleshas can be reduced through meditation.*

*We can learn to understand our fears/kleshas by observing the mind. These exist in our subconscious as well as in our conscious mind to varying degrees. In our normal daily state, we rarely see the character of the kleshas. We can not eliminate the kleshas with the help of the intellect; it can only be done with meditation.*

*It takes a sharp ability to pay attention to become aware of how kleshas look in ourselves. For example, we may believe that we are not afraid of death even though we unconsciously are. We do not see it. Even individuals who have been engaged in spiritual development for a long time – who for several years have experienced peace and thought they are free from samskaras and kleshas, can suddenly experience obstacles and failure. The kleshas' seed, root, and cause remain and come up to the surface. You need to practice the whole yoga system in-depth to eliminate kleshas. Yamas, niyamas and Kriya yoga.*

*By dhyana, i.e., to observe what happens to us mentally. It is done by paying attention to our good and bad thoughts and letting them surface. In the long run, it prevents kleshas from manifesting in the most active form, which creates suffering and fear in our daily lives. In this case, one does not refer to "object focus" when discussing dhyana but assumes mouna, i.e., one focuses on how kleshas look and its character and strength.*

*By focusing and observing, vrittis is weakened. It explains why meditation has such a calming effect on us. During meditation, our unconscious fears can surface so that we become aware of them. Tensions caused by our fears/kleshas are weakened, and we can relax. A feeling of inner harmony arises.*

*When our fears/kleshas have taken on a more latent form, we should, through our discernment / viveka, try to find the cause of the fear. You may be dependent on something, or you want to be successful.*

*Dhyana (Raja yoga) and Viveka (Jnana yoga) are thus two essential tools in eliminating our fears/kleshas. To prevent being drawn back to the unconscious state again – when one experiences risk becoming too challenging to deal with – Karma and Bhakti yoga can be beneficial.*

**2:1**

*What is yoga?*

**Yogaschitta vṛitti nirodhah**

*Yogah: yoga, chitta: consciousness, vritti: patterns, movements, nirodhah: blocked – still.*

*When the movements of the mind are still, yoga occurs.*

*Chitta refers to the mind, the individual consciousness on the conscious, unconscious, and subconscious planes.*

*Nirodhah aims to block the movements of the mind, the pattern of consciousness, not the mind or consciousness itself. It happens automatically when we sleep. The normal flow of vrittis is stopped, and we are moved to another state of consciousness. We experience other things, people, events, and places. With this, we can understand that within us, something exists independently of our body, mind, and life energy/prana, something utterly different from any of these. This "something" is consciousness, a constant and uninterrupted state.*

*Vritti can be translated as "circular," which describes chitta's movements. They are like rings on the water.*

*So, what is yoga? Yoga is to calm the movements of the mind on all planes of consciousness. It is not about shutting down or shielding oneself from the external impressions we encounter daily. We want to get past the experiences and visions that our consciousness creates during deep meditation and higher stages of samadhi. When this happens, yoga occurs. It is a prerequisite for the development of human consciousness.*

*When one ceases to identify with Prakriti, the three gunas develop our consciousness.*

*They talk about the five different characters of the mind. If you compare these with the Kundalini awakening, you can see that moodha / the sluggish mind is associated with the Mooladhara chakra, where the individual consciousness is dormant.*

*After practicing specific exercises, the consciousness is stimulated to direct itself to the area around the navel, the Manipura chakra. This state of consciousness is called kshipta and belongs to rajas. Most often, however, it sinks to Mooladhara chakra again and then rises to Swadhisthana chakra, Manipura chakra, and again to Mooladhara chakra. Once consciousness has stabilized in the Manipura chakra for some time – vikshipta, it will steer further through the Anahata chakra and the Vishuddhi chakra to the Ajna chakra. In this state of consciousness – echagrata, the consciousness is focused and concentrated, sattvic. Further, in the Sahasrara chakra, one achieves the state of nirodha beyond the three gunas and sattva.*

*The interaction between the three gunas governs all functions in our body, mind, and environment. Even though one guna dominates, the other two are always present and affect our consciousness. We should learn to see which guna dominates and how the other two come into play and then learn to balance these to control consciousness.*

**3:1**

*When yoga culminates – then the sight is established.*

**Tadā draṣṭuh svarūpe ́vasthānam**

*Tada: then, drasuh: seeing – answer, upe: the essential nature of oneself, vasthanam: establish, develop.*

*The seeing develops in its true nature.*

*Self-awareness, kaivalya, is the very goal of yoga in this context. It develops when the activity of chitta vritti ceases, when the mind is no longer affected by the interaction of the three gunas, and when one stops to identify with the material world.*

*The insight into our true nature comes from within. It is impossible to create or experience this insight in the state of consciousness where one still identifies with the self, the ego. Reaching this insight takes purity of mind, complete mind control, and freedom from desire.*

**4:1**

*What else happens to Purusha?*

**Vátti sārūpyamitaratra**

*Vrtti: modification, pattern, syrupy: identification, iterate: another state.*

*Otherwise, there is an identification with the movements of the mind.*

*When the movements of the mind, chitta vrittis, are not in the state of nirodha and have not calmed down, Purusha can not become aware of himself. Instead, there is an identification with chitta and its fluctuations.*

*When there is no awareness of the pure consciousness, Purusha, we identify with the movements of the chitta and are controlled by emotions such as feeling angry, sad, or scared.*

*Patanjali describes different techniques that are adapted to the different needs of individuals, depending on temperament, to lead chitta to the state of nirodha. It is a prerequisite for Purusha to become aware of its true nature.*

**5:1**

*Vrittis – main divisions.*

**Vṛttayah pañchatayyah kliṣṭāakliṣṭāh**

*Vrttayah: modification of the mind, pañchatayyah: fivefold, klista: painful, difficult, aklistah: not painful.*

*The modification of the mind is fivefold; these are either painful or not.*

*There are five types of vrittis, either painful or non-painful. In total, there are ten types of vrittis. When you experience something pleasant, e.g., looking at a beautiful flower, it is called aklishta. When you experience something painful and uncomfortable, it is called klishta.*

*According to Patanjali, everything we see, hear, think, and feel is a different formation of the mind. According to the yogic system, all our thoughts, knowledge, and various planes of consciousness are vital, as well as our dreams.*

**6:1**

*Five types of vrittis.*

**Pramāṇa-viparyaya-vikalpa-nidrā smṛtayah**

*Pramana: right knowledge, viparyaya: wrong knowledge,
vikalpa: imagination, nidra: sleep, smrtayah: memory.*

*The five different patterns of the mind are proper knowledge,
wrong knowledge, imagination, sleep, and memory.*

*Our mind comprises five types of vrittis: correct knowledge,
false knowledge, imagination, deep sleep, and memory. These
five build up the mind and shape the three dimensions of the
individual consciousness. All states of mind belong to these
five sensory patterns or vrittis (wakefulness, dreams, seeing,
speaking, hearing, touching, crying, feeling, and doing).*

*The ultimate goal of yoga is to break down these manifesta-
tions of the pattern of consciousness, i.e., vrittis.*

**12:1**

*The importance of abhyasa and vairagya.*

**Abhyāsavairāgyābhyām tannirodhah**

*Abhyasa: continuous practice, vairagyabhyam: through, vairagya, tat: it, nirodhah: stills.*

*Calming the five movement patterns of the mind takes place through regular exercise and vairagya.*

*Patanjali describes two ways to stop the flow of chitta vrittis. Abhyasa and vairagya. Abhyasa means regular exercise. Vairagya aims at liberation from raga and dweshta, i.e., attraction and reluctance to like/dislike. If you have control over these, meditation will be more accessible.*

**15:1**

*A lower state of vairagya.*

**Dṛṣṭānuśravika-viṣayāvitṛṣṇasya vaśīkāra-sañjñā vairāgyam**

*Drsta: the seen, anusravika: the heard, visaya: object, vitr-snasya: of the one free from desire, vasikara: control, sañjña: consciousness, vairagyam: absence of desire.*

*The state of consciousness is when the individual becomes free from the desire to satisfy the mind with what has previously been experienced, and what one has heard of is vairagya.*

*It is called vairagya when one is free from desire and no longer longs for the pleasures one has experienced. One is free from hunger in the face of all objects of the mind.*

*It is possible to achieve vairagya even if one lives in a normal society with a family and job. It is not necessary to give up these. However, what you absolutely must give up completely is raga and dweshta.*

*Vairagya starts from within ourselves, not from outside. It does not matter what clothes you wear or which people you live with. What matters is what kind of attitude you have towards the events and people you meet in life. Vairagya is divided into three stages. In the first step, you are fully aware of the desires and unwillingness that you carry, and you work to get over raga and dweshsta. In the second stage, some objects of raga and dwehsta have been taken over, but something remains. In the third stage, the mind is entirely free from these, but they can remain latent in the subconscious.*

**16:1**

*A higher state of vairagya.*

**Tatparam puruṣakhyāterguṇavaitṛṣṇyam**

*Tat: it, param: supreme, purusakhyateh: proper knowledge of Purusha, gunavaitrsnyam: free from the lusts of gunas.*

*The highest is when one becomes free from the lusts of gunas with the knowledge of Purusha.*

*Once one has reached this higher state of vairagya, there is no longer a need to experience pleasure and enjoyment, acquire knowledge, or be dependent on sleep. This state of vairagya is achieved when one becomes aware of Purusha.*

**21:1**

*The strength of curiosity is faster.*

**Tåvrasamveganamasannah**

*Tlvra: intensity, samvega: curiosity, asannah: close.*

*Those with intense curiosity and desire, samvega, achieve asamprajnata samadhi soon.*

*One realizes that everything is perishable, which is a prere-quisite for wanting to seek the truth.*

**23:1**

*The degree of curiosity and devotion to Ishwara (God).*

**Mṛdumadhyādhimātratvāt tato´pi viśeṣah**

*Mrdu: small, madhya: medium, adhimatra: strong, tvat: dependent on, tatopi: even, more than, viseah: specific.*

*As the desire grows in intensity from being minor to becoming strong, asamprajnata samadhi can be achieved faster. God refers to a superior spiritual consciousness. It is neither physical nor mental but only spiritual—the highest manifested consciousness in man. According to Patanjali, if you find it challenging to develop spiritually through the techniques described, you can also do so by devoting yourself intensely to God.*

**28:1**

*Sadhana for Ishvara.*

## Tajjapastadarthabhāvanam

*Tat: it, japa: repetition of the word, tat: it, artha: meaning, bhavanam: filled with mental.*

*To recite Aum and fill the mind with its meaning.*

*What separates Ishwara from man is that man is the manifested state of consciousness, while Ishwara is the highest state. The displayed condition continues to be manifested through rebirths and incarnations and takes shape in various bodies, such as humans and animals. It forms a finer and more developed body when it reaches the highest stage of evolution. Ishvara is beyond the manifestation of life and death and is, therefore, seen as the guru of the departed masters and prophets.*

*One must be able to reach Ishwara by thinking or speaking and by our intellect. Feeling and experiencing are two different things. The Indian philosophical system is divided into tattwa chintana, a reflection of the highest consciousness, and tattwa darshan, an experience of the highest consciousness. India's six intelligent systems are based on tattwa chintana, i.e., knowledge. Tattwa darshan's experience develops through yoga, Bhakti, mystery, and occult rituals.*

*Aum is like a means of expression for Ishwara, which is otherwise wholly formless. It is described in yantra, mantra, and Tantra. These three are expressions of the supernatural. Mantra is like a term in the form of sound. Pure consciousness is denoted and described in terms of the power of sound. In Tantra, there is symbolism in the form of humans and animals. Yantra is a mental symbol. Aum is both a mantra and a yantra. It is not Tantra, as it must have a human form and have no sound.*

*We cannot experience Ishwara with our eyes or ears, but we experience it within ourselves using a mantra. Aum denotes Ishvara.*

*The meditation becomes complete by constantly repeating the words Aum and dhyana about their meaning. Japa is not enough but must go hand in hand with meditation. Patanjali recommends that during the rehearsal of Aum, one should be aware of japa and its significance. Therefore, it is essential to understand the meaning of Aum. It is made up of three letters A-u-m. A relates to the world we perceive with our senses and body. U relates to the subconscious mind. M relates to the unconscious mind. By understanding this and repeating the mantra, one can change the three states of manifested consciousness, go beyond these, and finally reach the fourth and mysterious stage of consciousness called turiya, i.e., the unmanifest state of Purusha.*

**30-32:1**

*Obstacles that may appear during sadhana and how to get past them.*

*1. Disease.*
*2. Lethargy.*
*3. Well-being.*
*4. Lack of action.*
*5. Laziness.*
*6. Strong desires.*
*7. Wrong perception.*
*8. Instability.*
*9. Shaking.*
*10. Pain.*
*11. Depression.*

*Knowing and being prepared is essential; difficulties and obstacles are part of the sadhana's path. When the consciousness is turned inwards, the metabolism and functions of the body change. You may fall asleep during meditation or have different perceptual experiences.*

*The person often does not care about their personal life, family, and other chores. You may experience doubts and feel unsure if the sadhana is correct or you will reach the goal. You must focus on one principle – a mantra or a symbol to eliminate obstacles. One should, therefore, stick to a parti-*

cular mantra or symbol and not change it. Otherwise, the obstacles will become a fact.

There is no real difference between the symbols, but if you change the symbol, confusion is created in the mind.

**33:1**

*Creating Opposite Virtues - The Four Attitudes.*

**Maitrīkarunāmuditopeksānam sukhaduhkhapunyā-
punyaviṣayāṇām bhāvanātaśchittaprasādanam**

*Maitri: kindness, karuna: compassion, mudito: joy, upek-
sanam: indifference, sukha: happiness, duhkha: suffering,
punya: virtue, apunya: burden, visayanam: goal, bhavana-
tah: attitude, chitta: mind, prasadanam: pure.*

*To concentrate the mind, it must first be purified and stilled.
It is done by developing attitudes of kindness, compassion,
joy, indifference, and respect for individuals and events that
create happiness, suffering, virtues, or mistakes.*

*Through these attitudes, which are:*

*1. Friendship with the happy.*
*2. Compassion for the unfortunate.*
*3. Gratitude and joy for what goes well.*
*4. Indifference to what goes wrong.*

*It creates a calm and undisturbed mind. It is part of the
nature of the mind to be drawn to the outside world. It is not
part of the nature of the mind to look inward. When turning
the mind inward, one must first remove obstacles and impurities. These four attitudes remove these obstacles on both a
conscious and an unconscious level.*

**34:1**

*Control of prana.*

**Prachchhardanavidhāraṇābhyām vā prāṇasya**

*Prachchhardana: rechaka, vidharaan, bhyam: kumbakha, va: eller, pranasya; breathing.*

*By prolonging and keeping the spirit out, one can control the mind.*

*The whole mental structure consists of four different parts. Depending on the individual's temperament, different yoga paths fit differently.*

*1. Karma Yoga – dynamic people.*

*2. Bhakti yoga – emotional individuals.*

*3. Raya, Kriya, Swara yoga – psychic.*

*4. Jnana Yoga – intellectual persons.*

*We are often a mixture of all these and can benefit from practicing all paths. We should choose a sadhana that suits us best to create as little resistance as possible.*

*Patanjali describes pranayama and how we can calm our minds by keeping the spirit inside and out of the body* through three locks. He describes maha bandha, where you do jalandhara, uddiyana, and moola bandha while keeping your breath out. If you are a beginner, you can practice rechaka and kapalbhati to begin with.

With the help of these exercises, the mind is calmed. It is said that the mind has two supports: prana and vasana. These are supports on which the mind rests, and the consciousness works. If you delete one of these, the other also disappears automatically.

Pranan can be both rough and subtle. The subtle pran exists in the form of energy, and the coarse pran is our breathing.

There are five main prana vayu that we have touched on before: prana, apana, udana, samana, and vyana vayu. There are also five smaller pranas: devatta, nada, kurma, krikara and dhananjaya. All of these control different parts of the body's functions:

Prana controls our inhalation and acts in the mouth and nose, digests food, separates nutrients from food, converts the water in the body into sweat and urine, and controls the secretion of the glands. Its area is between the heart and the nose.

*The apana removes impurities and residues from the body and moves downward. Its area is around the navel and feet.*

*Samana works in our limbs and nadis. It acts in the area around the heart and navel.*

*Udana maintains our muscular strength and the energy that prevails when our karmic body leaves our physical body during death. It acts in the area around the neck and head.*

*Vyana controls blood circulation and moves through our nerves.*

*Nada controls coughing and sneezing, kurma controls contractions, krikara controls hunger and thirst, devatta creates drowsiness and sleep, and dhananjaya maintains nutrition.*

*There are also fine channels in the body called nadis. Prana/ impulses and signals flow to and from the brain through these. In total, we have about seventy-two thousand different nadis.*

*Ida, pingala, and sushuman are the three most important nadis, of which sushumna is the most crucial channel for spiritual consciousness. These three start from the Mooladhara chakra and meet in the Ajna chakra.*

*Our breathing controls our thoughts in the present, past, and future. During the day, breathing alternates through the right and left nostrils. You usually breathe for one hour through the right nostril and then one hour through the left nostril and about twelve times a day through each. The left nostril is called the ida, and the right is the pingala. When the breathing changes from pingala to ida or from ida to pingala, the sushumna flows temporarily.*

*Performing heavy work is best suited when pingala nadi is flowing. When ida nadi flows, lighter work is best done. When sushumna nadi flows, meditation is best suited. We can control the flow through the nostrils with the help of various exercises.*

**35:1**

*Pay attention to sensory experiences.*

**Viṣayavatī vā pravṛttirutpannā manasah sthitiniband-
hanī**

*Visayavati: sensual, va: or, pravrttih: functioning, panning:
arises, manasah: of the mind, sthiti: steadfastness, nibandha-
ni: which binds.*

*The mind can be made steady by keeping it active with sen-
sory experiences.*

*Suppose you experience Ishwara pranidhara, maha bandha,
or pranayama, which is challenging to practice. In that case,
you can instead use different sensory experiences such as
sight, hearing, smell, taste, and touch to create a steady and
calm mind.*

*Nada yoga (antar mouna).*
*Trataka.*
*Kirtan.*
*Mantra.*

**36:1**

*Experience the inner light – optional meditation on what the mind is drawn to naturally.*

**Viśokā vā jyotiṣmatī**

*Visoka: without sorrow, va: or, jyotismati: filled with light.*

*When filled with light, the state beyond grief can control the mind.*

*The mind can also be stilled by experiencing the inner calm and the clear white light between the eyebrows – bhrumadhya or through nada, concentration on sound. This inner glow is calm, still, and peaceful and is experienced during deep meditation when you are sattvic, and Kundalini Shakti flows through the sushumna and activates all your chakras. The sound is spandam – aum, the sound of creation and comsos; you hear it as a beeping sound of Bindu slowly increasing in power. When you see the light and hear the sound, you are connected. You send, and you receive the intensity of the cosmos. You are one with the universe's intelligence, the collective consciousness – God.*

# MEDITATION

*Meditation aims to establish contact with his inner self and increase his self-awareness. The goal is to realize oneself. When a person achieves self-realization, they communicate with their innermost self and identify their existence – their life, based on their true self and not based on their ego. During meditation, one tries to establish an observed self, which means studying one's thoughts objectively and neutrally. Thus, gaining a perspective on one's thoughts, feelings, and existence is necessary.*

*The purpose of meditation is to explore the different regions of the mind, learn how the mind works, and train it to surpass the mind finally. In practical terms, meditation is about emptying the mind of thoughts by concentrating on the present through an activity or method.*

## ACTIVE MEDITATION

*Active meditation means breathing with some form of movement to calm the thoughts and get into the present. Examples of active meditation are yoga, qigong, and tai chi. Dynamic meditation can also be part of our everyday life through walks, eating, etc. if you do it with the presence of putting your feet up and breathing. How it feels in the body, etc.*

**PASSIVE MEDITATION**

*Passive meditation – which most people may associate with meditation- means you are silent to practice some meditation techniques. One trains the mind through a specific method or process to put oneself in a meditative state.*

*Unlike in the past, research has recently begun to look at the holistic aspect of man a little more. Research on meditation has increased enormously. The reason for this may be the increased mental disorders and diseases that are today a public health problem in many countries. The current research that has been done on yoga and meditation shows clear and measurable results on stress-related issues such as neck and back problems, headaches, depression, anxiety, weight problems, and difficulty sleeping.*

*To overcome these mental problems, meditation has become an increasingly recommended and used method. More and more psychologists today advise their clients to practice meditation to connect with their inner self and emotions, for example. Psychology has now come to believe that the regular stage of a human being is a constant joy.*

*In research on meditation, pulsating electrical voltages are measured, which the brain gives rise to so-called brain waves. These brain waves are measured via EEG (Electro Encephalo Gram: electric-brain registration). These waves can display different frequencies, which are divided into four stages. The first stage is called beta waves and is the one we have during normal waking. Alpha waves are the second stage, and we are then relaxed and have a milder state of mind than meditation. We have theta waves when we dream. Conversely, children may be in this stage when awake, but it is less common in adults. Delta waves are likened to deep sleep (without dreams). An experienced yogi can go from beta waves to delta waves during meditation. Research has also shown that those who have practiced meditation for a long time have more stable brain waves (have constant coherence) and a more excellent mental balance, i.e., triggers endorphins that strengthen the immune system.*

*Physiologically, meditation reduces muscle tension, improves respiratory rhythm, digestion, immune system, blood pressure, and heart rate, and increases the efficiency of the internal organs.*

*Many people who meditate regularly experience that they get more energy, become more alert, and sleep better; the stress level in the body decreases, concentration and the ability to focus are strengthened, and the ability to perform and oxygen uptake is improved.*

*The autonomic nervous system is divided into the sympathetic nervous system and the parasympathetic nervous system.*

*The sympathetic nervous system is usually called the "fight or flight defense system," which is the system that is activated during mental or physical stress. When this is activated, the pupils dilate, blood pressure increases, digestion decreases, and blood sugar increases. The parasympathetic nervous system is the opposite, starting when the body is at rest. It lowers blood pressure, stimulates digestion, improves healing processes, and secretes oxytocin (the body's calm and growth hormone). These two systems complement each other.*

*Today's society and our lives result in the sympathetic nervous system being activated in many people almost all the time. The sympathetic nervous system is meant to be activated only for short periods. Still, as today's threats often consist of fears of being unable to pay bills, worries about the job, etc., they often become activated for longer. It leads to people always being tense, unhappy, and having a more challenging time resisting illness. If the sympathetic nervous system is activated, it can also lead to high blood pressure, diabetes, heart attack, and several mental disorders linked to stress.*

*The only way to prevent this is through physical and mental relaxation and, of course, with good sleep. Meditation provides both physical and psychological relaxation. We must also learn to react differently to our surroundings and what we are exposed to daily so that the adrenaline content only sometimes increases.*

**THINKING ABOUT MEDITATION**

*When sitting down for meditation, thinking about a few things is essential. The first preparation is that you can sit undisturbed, where you feel silent. Turn off all phones and make sure no one is disturbed. The morning or before bedtime are the best times for meditation. Also, remember not to eat too close to the meditation, as the body is full of digestion, and a lot of blood and energy is drawn in from the body to the stomach. Ensure you have done yoga or exercised before so that all restlessness is out of your body. Ensure your signal systems are balanced by asanas so that Kundalini Shakti can flow freely in the sushumna nadi and activate your chakras on the way up to the Sahasrara chakra.*

*Then, ensure you have something to sit on: a meditation pillow, a regular pillow, or a chair. Take the time to find a comfortable sitting position. It would help if you sat comfortably as you will sit still for a while. A popular sitting position is siddhasana, where you sit on the buttocks with the legs outstretched, insert one foot towards the groin, and place the other foot just in front of the shin or on top of the shin. Make sure you are sitting in a three-point position where both buttocks are in contact with the ground and both knees.*

*You place your hands on your knees with the palm facing down and let your thumb and forefinger meet in jnana mudra. Alternatively, place the proper back of the hand in the left palm and let the thumbs meet in bhairavi mudra. It is essential that you feel your hands resting securely so that you can relax your shoulders.*

*Feel that you are sitting with a straight spine where the weight from the upper body can fall straight down through the pelvis. Insert your chin slightly next to your chest so your neck can relax and close your eyes. Have a little weight forward on the pelvis so you do not collapse with your back.*

*Then start by landing in yourself with your thoughts and presence, calm the mind, and relax the body with kaya stahairyam. Then begin your chosen meditation technique with, for example, ajapa japa. It is essential not to have any expectations of the meditation and what one is believed to experience.*

*There are also various obstacles that one may encounter during meditation, such as thoughts and feelings. There can be obstacles such as anger, pride, and selfishness, which can be trained away, among other things. Practice yamas and niyamas. If any ideas or feelings arise during the meditation, become aware of them, see them, but then let them float on with the next exhalation and then return to focusing on the chosen meditation technique.*

*When the mind is still, and you are sattvic, the white light between the eyebrows – bhrumadhya, slowly emerges. Kundalini Shakti flows through the sushumna nadi, and all your chakras are activated. You hear a beeping sound from Bindu, which is gradually increasing power. When you see the light and hear the sound, you are connected.*

*If it is difficult to calm down, it can be advantageous to have done something active before setting out for meditation, such as taking a walk or doing a yoga session.*

*It is essential to have regularity in your meditation practice.*

## CLASSICAL TECHNIQUES FOR MEDITATION

*The classic sitting positions for meditation (meditation asanas) are padmasana, siddhasana, siddha yoni asana, and swastikasana. For beginners (and Westerners who are often stiff and have narrower hips), you can also sit in sukhasana or ardha padmasana. You can do so if you need to sit on a chair for various reasons. The principle is that the sitting position should be comfortable and support the body during meditation so you can relax. It's about something other than sitting nicely. The back must be straight so that the prana can flow upwards in the body. You can also lie comfortably on your back, but then there is the risk of falling asleep.*

*Important mudras during meditation include jnana/chin mudra, bhairavi mudra, and khechari mudra.*

## JNANA MUDRA

*Place your hands on your knees with your palms facing down, and let your thumb and forefinger meet.*

## CHIN MUDRA

*Place your hands on your knees with the palm facing up, and let your thumb and forefinger meet.*

## BHAIRAVI MUDRA

*You place the proper back of the hand in the left palm and let your thumbs meet.*

## KHECHARI MUDRA

*Roll up the tongue so that you place the back of the tongue up in the palate with gentle pressure.*

## UJJAYI PRANAYAMA

*Ujjayi pranayama is also called the psychic/winning breath. Start by placing the back of the tongue up in the palate in the khechari mudra, narrow in the air passage, and strive for a whispering/hissing – "ah" sound. Breathe through your nose, but feel that the breathing and the sound come far in from the throat. It sounds like when you blow mist on a mirror with an open mouth. Children usually say that the sound is similar to Darth Vader's breathing in Star Wars.*

*Ujjayi pranayama is used in many different meditation tech-*

niques (and also during the practice of asanas) as it calms the nervous system and lowers blood pressure. It also emits a sound as a focal point to draw attention to. Breathing in this way also means that you retain the heat.

## BHRUMADHYA

Bhrumadhya is a trigger point for the Ajna chakra (third eye). The word bhrumadhya means eyebrow center, also where this point is located.

## CHIDAKASHA

Chidakasha can be explained as our inner mental television screen. It is visualized as space before our closed eyes, where our psychic event/event appears – "what the mind carries." Chidakasha stands for "area of knowledge," and Akasha means space—our microcosmos.

## JAPA YOGA

Using the mantra, Japa yoga is an effective technique for returning the mind to the present. Japa means repetition of a mantra. The mantra affects us physically and mentally with the help of the word's meaning and vibrations within one. Mantra meditation cleanses the subconscious mind and causes the thought activity to decrease, as the mind does not receive any new stimulus. It makes it easier to get in touch with your inner self.

*Constantly repeating the mantra makes the mind concentrated and relaxed and gives us inner peace. It is important not to force focus on the mantra but to let it come naturally from within. One can practice japa with different forms of mantras; it can be mantras that one pronounces aloud (baikhari), mantras to whisper (upanshu), mental mantras (mansaik), or written mantras (likhit). You often recite the mantra a certain number of times, and to help you with the count, you can have a mala, a rosary with pearls. You can practice Japa yoga while sitting in a meditation position and performing other daily activities. If you are rajasic, you should be careful not to increase the tempo of the mantra or become stressed by it.*

## AJAPA JAPA

*Ajapa japa is a complete sadhana (spiritual practice where one eventually achieves self-realization). By regularly practicing ajapa japa for a long time, subconscious desires and fears will finally come to the surface, which one will then view with a witness attitude and thus get to the root of physical and mental problems and can change them.*

*Japa means repetition of a mantra. Ajapa japa means constant awareness. Traditionally, the mantra So-Ham is used, but it is possible to use any mantra if, for example, you have received a mantra from your guru.*

## HARI OM TAT SAT

*A guided meditation often ends with Hari Om Tat Sat in classical yoga.*


*Hari Om and Tat Sat are two different mantras brought together; Hari Om is one, and Tat Sat is the other. Hari stands for the manifested universe and life, the energy – Shakti. Om stands for the absolute reality, the consciousness – Shiva. Reality consists of the complete (incomprehensible) and the obvious / the more concrete. This reality is presented in the mantra Hari Om Tat Sat. Satya means truth. Tat Sat means "it is the truth." Hari Om Tat Sat means both the concrete – what I can see and the unknown or incomprehensible, which is also part of the same reality and not different.*

# YOGASCHITTA VRITTI NIRODHAH

## (WHEN THE MOVEMENTS OF THE MIND ARE STILL, YOGA OCCURS)

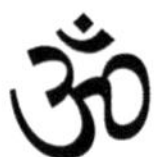

*Did you like the book? Feel free to follow me on my social media, share and like, tell your friends about the books, and feel free to write an honest review; one or two lines don't matter. All support is precious. Thanks!*

*On my Facebook page and Instagram, I post exciting news and tips on temporary offers and benefits you can take advantage of. I often also post my yoga routine and other things related to nutrition and health that may be interesting to take part in. So feel free to join them so you don't miss anything interesting:*

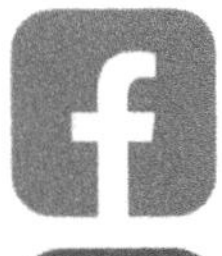 *facebook.com/bhagwanoneofakindbooks*

 *instagram.com/bhagwanoneofakindbooks/*

## MY BOOKS AND BOOK SERIES

*I have two book series that have different audiences. Great Yoga Books – is a series with the most comprehensive fact books on yoga for those who want to explore the subject in depth. Here, you will also find classic yoga books that are rarely translated, such as Patanjali's Yoga Sutras and Hatha Yoga Pradipika. My second series, Yoga Beyond the Poses: The Ultimate Beginner's Guide to Yoga, covers one yoga topic at a time and is extra easy to read with larger text. For those who find it challenging to read extensive books and want a good and broad overview of the subject quickly. Both series are also available as audiobooks.*

★★★★★

# TEACHING YOGA
# &
# MEDITATION
# BEYOND
# THE POSES

## BESTSELLING AUTHOR

# Shreyananda
# Natha

**Teaching Yoga and Meditation Beyond the Poses – A unique and practical workbook!**

*Teaching Yoga and Meditation Beyond the Poses – A unique and practical workbook for aspiring yoga teachers who want to teach yoga and meditation beyond the poses.*

*Teaching Yoga and Meditation Beyond the Poses is a unique and essential resource for new and experienced teachers and a guide for all yoga students interested in refining their skills and knowledge. Teaching Yoga and Meditation is also ideal as a core textbook in yoga teacher training programs.*

*The book covers fundamental yoga philosophy and history topics, including a historical presentation of classical yoga literature: Yoga Sutras of Patanjali, Bhagavad Gita, etc. Each of the seven major styles of yoga is described, from Hatha yoga, Raja yoga, Tantra yoga, Bhakti yoga, and Kundalini yoga, to knowledge about the chakras, Ayurveda and magic mantras and yantras. The book provides extensive support and tools for teaching integrated and classical yoga (asanas), breathing techniques (pranayama), deep relaxation (Yoga Nidra), and meditation (Ajapa Japa). The book is divided into eight modules with associated knowledge tests and complete yoga and meditation classes.*

https://rb.gy/9s6edj

*Download the* ***AUDIOBOOK*** *here!*

*SCAN QR-CODE or go to:*

***https://bit.ly/3Rf7Mpu***

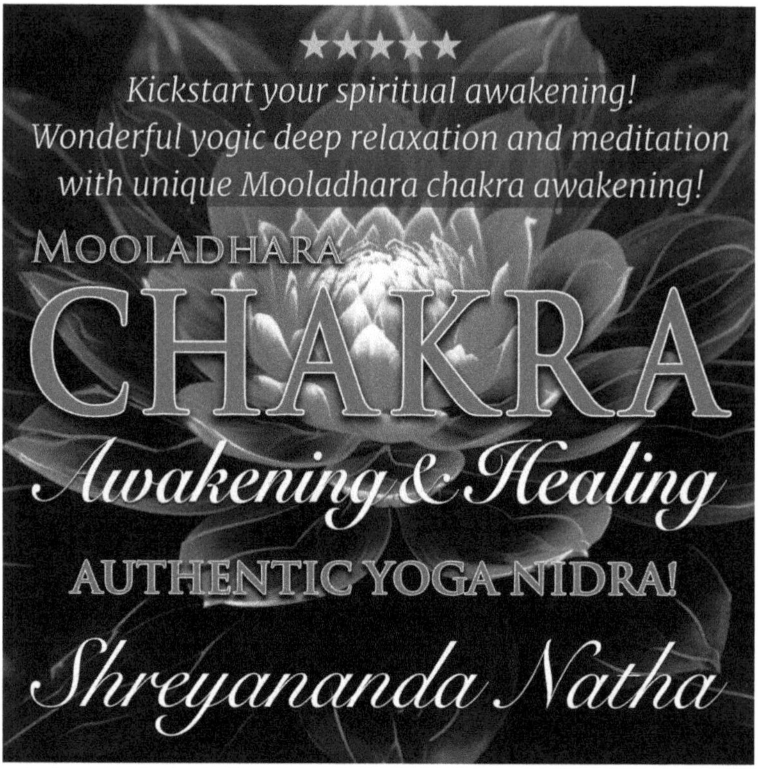